91 Natural Skin Cancer Juice and Meal Recipes:

Protect and Revive Your Skin Using Nutrient-Rich Ingredients

By

Joe Correa CSN

COPYRIGHT

This publication is designed to provide accurate and authoritative information in regard to the subject matter covered. It is sold with the understanding that neither the author nor the publisher is engaged in rendering medical advice. If medical advice or assistance is needed, consult with a doctor. This book is considered a guide and should not be used in any way detrimental to your health. Consult with a physician before starting this nutritional plan to make sure it's right for you.

ACKNOWLEDGEMENTS

This book is dedicated to my friends and family that have had mild or serious illnesses so that you may find a solution and make the necessary changes in your life.

91 Natural Skin Cancer Juice and Meal Recipes:

Protect and Revive Your Skin Using Nutrient-Rich Ingredients

By

Joe Correa CSN

CONTENTS

ABOUT THE AUTHOR

After years of Research, I honestly believe in the positive effects that proper nutrition can have over the body and mind. My knowledge and experience has helped me live healthier throughout the years and which I have shared with family and friends. The more you know about eating and drinking healthier, the sooner you will want to change your life and eating habits.

Nutrition is a key part in the process of being healthy and living longer so get started today. The first step is the most important and the most significant.

INTRODUCTION

91 Natural Skin Cancer Juice and Meal Recipes: Protect and Revive Your Skin Using Nutrient-Rich Ingredients

By Joe Correa CSN

This book includes the best skin cancer preventive juices available to ensure your skin is strong and healthy in the least amount of time. Juicing is fast way to absorb essential cancer-fighting vitamins and minerals your body needs to protect itself from harmful toxins.

When it comes to preventing skin cancer, you might focus only on using sunscreen, a hat, long-sleeve shirts, or staying in the shade but you can still do much more. A diet rich in cancer-fighting vitamins and minerals can make a world of a difference when trying to prevent skin cancer.

To prevent and treat skin cancer it's crucial to maintain a healthy lifestyle (no alcohol, no smoking, doing exercise regularly and if possible outdoors, etc.) and a well-balanced diet. When trying to prevent or treat skin cancer, good eating habits can significantly reduce your chances of getting cancer or may at least help slow melanoma progression.

Foods rich in antioxidants, vitamins A, B, C, and D, and other compounds such as carotenoids, (especially beta-carotene) have proven to have many anti-carcinogenic properties that help to keep skin healthy and beautiful.

COMMITMENT

In order to improve my condition, I *(your name)*, commit to eating more of these foods on a daily basis and to exercise at least 30 minutes daily:

- Berries (especially blueberries), peaches, cherries, apples, apricots, oranges, lemon juice, grapefruit, tangerines, mandarins, pears, etc.
- Broccoli, spinach, collard greens, sweet potatoes, avocado, artichoke, baby corn, carrots, celery, cauliflower, onions, etc.
- Whole grains, steel-cut oats, oatmeal, quinoa, barley, etc.
- Black beans, red bean beans, garbanzo beans, lentils, etc.
- Nuts and seeds including: walnuts, cashews, flaxseeds, sesame seeds, etc.
- Fish
- 8 – 10 glasses of water

Sign here

X_____

91 NATURAL SKIN CANCER JUICE AND MEAL RECIPES: PROTECT AND REVIVE YOUR SKIN USING NUTRIENT-RICH INGREDIENTS

JUICES

1.   PROTECTOR JUICE

In this juice, you will enjoy the perks of carotenoids such as alpha and beta-carotene found in carrots and the interactions of its components that make carrots a highly recommended vegetable for the prevention of many types of cancers such as skin cancer.

Ingredients:

- 2 Carrots, peeled
- 1 Apple
- 1 Celery stalk
- 1 tsp honey
- 1 cup water

Instructions:

- ✓ Wash the carrots, apple and celery stalk.

✓ Place all ingredients in a blender.

✓ Blend together while adding water until the desired consistency is reached.

2.   C+ POWER

Citric fruits are high in Vitamin C and other compounds that give them antioxidant properties. Also Vitamin C can reduce the negative sunburn reaction to UVB radiation, thus increasing the natural protective capabilities of our skin.

Ingredients:

- 1 cup Water
- 1 cup Green tea
- 1 Tamarillo
- ½ tsp Turmeric

Instructions:

- ✓ Wash tamarillo.
- ✓ Place all ingredients in a blender.
- ✓ Blend together while adding water until the desired consistency is reached.

3.   HYDRAJUICE

Green tea has many perks as it is well known for its antioxidant properties. Green tea contains catechins and other polyphenols, which have been related with anti-cancer properties and being able to protect your system from carcinogenic mutations.

Ingredients:

- 2 cups Green tea
- 1 cup diced watermelon
- 1 cup diced cantaloupe
- ¼ tsp ginger

Instructions:

- ✓ Place all ingredients in a blender.
- ✓ Blend together while adding water until the desired consistency is reached.

4.   BERRYLICIOUS

Blueberries and Raspberries are on the top of the list among antioxidants and anti-carcinogenic fruits; they have shown to contain a large variety of potent antitumor effects against cancer.

Ingredients:

- 2 cups Raspberries
- 1 cup Blueberries
- 2 Bananas
- 1 tsp cacao powder
- 2 cups coconut water

Instructions:

- ✓ Place all ingredients in a blender.
- ✓ Blend together while adding water until the desired consistency is reached.

5. TROPIJUICY

Avocados are a great source of healthy omega-3 fatty acids, which are known to have anti-inflammatory properties and have been related to protective effects against cancer. Research also suggests that omega 3 fatty acids can help protect the skin from UV damage.

Ingredients:

- 1 Avocado, pitted and peeled
- 1 cup cherries, pitted
- 1 tsp cacao powder
- 1 tbsp coconut flakes
- 1 cup coconut water

Instructions:

- ✓ Place all ingredients in a blender.
- ✓ Blend together while adding water until the desired consistency is reached.

6.   VITALITY JUICE

Watercress is a good source of various vitamins like A, B and C vitamins. It has also been shown that Watercress reduces cancer risk, increases immune function, reduces blood cell DNA damage and has great antioxidant properties that will protect your skin from carcinogenic effects.

Ingredients:

- 2 cups Watercress
- ½ Cucumber
- 1 cup Strawberries
- 1 cup water

Instructions:

- ✓ Wash watercress and cucumber.
- ✓ Place all ingredients in a blender.
- ✓ Blend together while adding water until the desired consistency is reached.

7. BERRY POWER

Grapes are highly recommended as they're a good source of resveratrol, which is a powerful antioxidant and is thought to help stop the aging process in humans, making them an excellent source for anti-cancer effects.

Ingredients:

- 1 cup Grapes
- 1 cup Raspberries
- ½ cup Pomegranate juice
- 1 cup diced Watermelon
- 1 cup water

Instructions:

- ✓ Wash grapes and raspberries.
- ✓ Place all ingredients in a blender.
- ✓ Blend together while adding water until the desired consistency is reached.

8. SUPERKALE

Among the cruciferous vegetables, kale has the highest levels of vitamins. It is also a good source of carotenoids and phytonutrients which have been reported to have anti-cancer properties.

Ingredients:

- 2 cups Kale
- 1 cup diced Pineapple
- ¼ cup of Basil
- ½ cup lemon juice
- 1 cup water

Instructions:

- ✓ Wash kale leaves.
- ✓ Place all ingredients in a blender.
- ✓ Blend together while adding water until the desired consistency is reached.

9.   WILD-O-RADISH BOOSTER

The family of brassica vegetables is vast and horseradish is one of its members, as well as broccoli and kale. This family of vegetables is well-known for having components with cancer preventive properties.

Ingredients:

- 2 radish, sliced
- ½ cup broccoli head, chopped
- ½ cup kale
- 1 cup Pomegranate juice
- ¼ cup almonds

Instructions:

- ✓ Wash radish, broccoli and kale.
- ✓ Place all ingredients in a blender.
- ✓ Blend together while adding water until the desired consistency is reached.

10. SUPER BERRYOCCOLI JUICE

Broccoli is highly recommended for a wide range of cancer and cardiovascular diseases. It's a good source of vitamins and substances that have been demonstrated for cancer-fighting properties and antioxidant protection.

Ingredients:

- 2 cup Broccoli heads, chopped
- 1 cup Blueberries
- 2 cups Grapefruit juice

Instructions:

- ✓ Wash blueberries and broccoli
- ✓ Place all ingredients in a blender.
- ✓ Blend together while adding water until the desired consistency is reached.

11. MEGA-D

For this juice we want to enhance the properties of cherries by using Greek Yogurt, a natural source of vitamin D. There has been a lot of research on the relation between skin cancer and vitamin D., indicating that lower levels of vitamin D can be related to an increased risk of developing melanoma so let's boost up with the MEGA-D juice.

Ingredients:

- 2 cups Cherries
- 1 large Banana, peeled
- 2 dates
- 1 cup Greek Yoghurt

Instructions:

- ✓ Wash cherries.
- ✓ Place all ingredients in a blender.
- ✓ Blend together while adding water until the desired consistency is reached.

12.   SPICY JUICY

Spinach contains various carotenoids and lignans which have anti-carcinogenic properties. Add the cucurbitacins found in cucumbers that also provide anticancer effects, and this makes this juice highly recommended to keep your body hydrated and also prevent melanoma.

Ingredients:

- 2 cups Baby spinach leaves
- 1 cucumber, sliced
- ½ cup lemon juice
- 1 cup water
- ¼ tsp hot pepper

Instructions:

- ✓ Wash the cucumber and spinach.
- ✓ Place all ingredients in a blender.
- ✓ Blend together while adding water until the desired consistency is reached.

13.   LYCOPENE BOOSTER

Tomatoes are full of goodness; they have shown to have antioxidant, anti-inflammatory, and cardio-protective properties. Several studies have found that greater consumption of tomatoes is associated with increased protection against sunburn and healthier skin.

Ingredients:

- 2 Tomatoes
- 1 Celery stalk
- 2 cups cranberry juice
- ¼ tsp Turmeric

Instructions:

- ✓ Wash the tomatoes and celery stalk.
- ✓ Place all ingredients in a blender.
- ✓ Blend together while adding water until the desired consistency is reached.

14.   MELON MIX

The consumption of these melons -watermelon, cantaloupe, honeydew, - boost your system due to the high amount of carotenoids, which can help protect your skin against harmful ultraviolet radiation from the sun.

Ingredients:

- 1 cup diced Cantaloupe
- 1 cup diced Watermelon
- 1 cup diced Honeydew
- 1 cup water
- 1 tsp of lemon juice

Instructions:

- ✓ Place all ingredients in a blender.
- ✓ Blend together while adding water until the desired consistency is reached.

15. PINK JUICE

Guavas are a great source of beta-carotene and Vitamin C. Research has proven their chemopreventive effects, and also they are delicious, being one of the best fruits to start adding to your skin cancer preventive diet.

Ingredients:

- 2 Guavas, peeled
- 1 large Banana, peeled
- ½ cup cherries, pitted
- ½ cup strawberries
- 1 cup water

Instructions:

- ✓ Wash cherries and strawberries.
- ✓ Place all ingredients in a blender.
- ✓ Blend together while adding water until the desired consistency is reached.

16.   APRICOT SUNRISE

In this juice you can enjoy the benefits of carotenoids as well as vitamin D and selenium, a compound related to reducing the risk of developing melanoma.

Ingredients:

- 2 cups Apricot slices
- 1 large banana, peeled
- ½ cup rolled oats
- 1 cup almond milk
- 3 tbsp Greek yogurt

Instructions:

- ✓ Place all ingredients in a blender.
- ✓ Blend together while adding water until the desired consistency is reached.

17.   PURPLE BOOSTER

Pomegranates are an excellent source of chemopreventive compounds thanks to their polyphenols and lignans as these compounds are capable of inhibiting carcinogenic cells.

Ingredients:

- 1 cup Pomegranate juice
- 2 cups Grapes, seedless
- 1 cup Blueberries

Instructions:

- ✓ Wash grapes and berries.
- ✓ Place all ingredients in a blender.
- ✓ Blend together while adding water until the desired consistency is reached.

18.   SELENIUMIGHTY

Brazil nuts are among the greatest sources for Selenium. This mineral helps you protect your skin from sunburns, due to its properties to create antioxidant enzymes. Selenium also boosts the effectiveness of Vitamin C found in Kiwifruit.

Ingredients:

- ½ cup Brazil nuts
- 1 Banana, peeled
- 1 Kiwifruit, washed and sliced
- 1 Fig
- 1 cup water

Instructions:

- ✓ Place all ingredients in a blender.
- ✓ Blend together while adding water until the desired consistency is reached.

19.   BETA-DRINK

Mustard greens are a natural source of important nutrients as it contains beta-carotene, vitamin A, vitamin C, calcium and iron. It especially has high contents of beta-carotene, the well-known skin protector.

Ingredients:

- 1 cup Mustard greens
- 1 cup chopped Mango
- ½ cup cherries
- 1 tsp lemon juice
- 1 cup water

Instructions:

- ✓ Wash mustard greens and cherries.
- ✓ Place all ingredients in a blender.
- ✓ Blend together while adding water until the desired consistency is reached.

20. GREEN ENERGY

Romaine lettuce is one of the most nutritious among all the lettuces. It contains great amounts of beta-carotene, lutein and vitamin K.

Ingredients:

- 2 cups Romaine Lettuce
- 1 Cucumber, sliced
- 1 cup chopped Pineapple
- 1 tsp lemon juice
- 1 cup water

Instructions:

- ✓ Wash romaine lettuce and cucumber.
- ✓ Place all ingredients in a blender.
- ✓ Blend together while adding water until the desired consistency is reached.

21. SUNSET JUICE

The compounds that give the orange-yellowish common coloration of apricots, peaches and pumpkins also provide anti-carcinogenic properties. Combine this with the many properties of turmeric, such as antioxidant, anti-inflammatory, and antibacterial effects, and you have a wonderful juice to prevent cancer.

Ingredients:

- 1 cup pumpkin purée
- 1 cup chopped peach
- 1 cup chopped apricot
- ½ tsp turmeric
- 1 cup water
- 4 walnuts, chopped

Instructions:

- ✓ Place all ingredients in a blender.
- ✓ Blend together while adding water until the desired consistency is reached.

22. BROBOOST

In this smoothie we are combining so much power. We will find Bromelain properties from the pineapples, plus carotenoids and antioxidants from spinach. All of these compounds give your body a great source of anti-cancer nutrients.

Ingredients:

- 1 cup chopped Pineapple fruit
- 2 cups Baby Spinach leaves
- ½ tsp ginger
- 1 cup water

Instructions:

- ✓ Wash the baby spinach leaves.
- ✓ Place all ingredients in a blender.
- ✓ Blend together while adding water until the desired consistency is reached.

23.   K+AID

Flaxseeds have a substantial amount of healthy omega-3 fatty acids. As cancer-preventive compounds, these healthy omega-3 fatty acids play an important role in regulating our immune system, which is a valuable role when aiming to prevent carcinogenic cells appearing in our bodies.

Ingredients:

- ½ cup flaxseeds
- 1 cup chopped apricots
- 1 Green apple, sliced
- 1 cup water

Instructions:

- ✓ Wash the green apple.
- ✓ Place all ingredients in a blender.
- ✓ Blend together while adding water until the desired consistency is reached.

24.　JUICYMINT

Let's highlight the benefits of raspberries: they are an incredible source of diverse phytochemicals, including ellagic acid and anthocyanin, both of which have shown to inhibit cancer cell growth.

Ingredients:

- 1 cup Raspberries
- 1 banana, peeled
- ¼ tsp Mint leaves
- 1 cup water

Instructions:

- ✓ Wash the raspberries.
- ✓ Place all ingredients in a blender.
- ✓ Blend together while adding water until the desired consistency is reached.

25.   ORIENTAL JUICE

Watermelon is also highly recommended for skin cancer prevention, because is an excellent source of carotenoids, L-citrulline, and cucurbitacins. These compounds have been shown to have chemopreventive properties so we have a delicious and nutritious juice.

Ingredients:

- 1 cup cubed watermelon
- 1 Kiwi, peeled, cubed
- 1 cup Green Tea
- 1 tsp honey

Instructions:

- ✓ Wash kiwi then peel and cube.
- ✓ Place all ingredients in a blender.
- ✓ Blend together while adding water until the desired consistency is reached.

26.   JUPITER BERRIES

Berries rank among the highest of all fruits and vegetables in their properties against cancer. Blueberries have amazing properties, including the ability to destroy free radicals, and to show neuroprotective and cardioprotective properties.

Ingredients:

- 1 cup Strawberries
- 1 cup Blueberries
- 1 cup Cherries
- 1 cup water

Instructions:

- ✓ Wash all the berries.
- ✓ Place all ingredients in a blender.
- ✓ Blend together while adding water until the desired consistency is reached.

27.   YELLOWISH

Turmeric has so many benefits as an antioxidant, anti-inflammatory, antibacterial, neuroprotective and cardio-protective compound. Some research has also shown that turmeric has a variety of anti-cancer properties against a wide range of cancers.

Ingredients:

- ½ tsp turmeric
- 1 cup chopped Papaya
- 1 cup chopped Mango
- 1 tsp lemon juice
- 1 cup water

Instructions:

- ✓ Place all ingredients in a blender.
- ✓ Blend together while adding water until the desired consistency is reached.

28.   LIFE-ENHANCING

Mangos are full of vitamins and beta-carotene, while blueberries and raspberries are well-known for its phytochemicals compounds that give them excellent anti-cancer properties.

Ingredients:

- 1 cup Mango slices
- 1 cup cherries, pitted
- 1 Fig
- 1 cup Broccoli florets
- 1 cup water

Instructions:

- ✓ Wash the cherries and broccoli florets.
- ✓ Place all ingredients in a blender.
- ✓ Blend together while adding water until the desired consistency is reached.

29.   HOLY JUICE

Pineapples have a unique compound which is been reported to have many anti-cancer properties called bromelain. This compound has pro-apoptic, anti-invasive and anti-metastatic properties so very useful in preventing skin cancer.

Ingredients:

- 2 cups chopped pineapple
- 1 green apple
- ½ sliced cucumber
- ½ tsp Ginger
- 1 cup water

Instructions:

- ✓ Wash the cucumber and apple.
- ✓ Place all ingredients in a blender.
- ✓ Blend together while adding water until the desired consistency is reached.

30. GRAN-AID

Research shows the anti-carcinogenic properties of pomegranate, as it is shown to inhibit the growth of skin cancer tumors. It also has chemopreventive properties so drinking pomegranate juice often can help stay away from skin cancer.

Ingredients:

- 2 cups chopped Honeydew
- 1 Kiwi, sliced
- 1 cup Pomegranate juice

Instructions:

- ✓ Wash kiwi then slice.
- ✓ Place all ingredients in a blender.
- ✓ Blend together while adding water until the desired consistency is reached.

31. SWISSBOOST

Swiss chard is one of the healthiest vegetables available. It is a terrific source of antioxidants and anti-inflammatory compounds such as beta-carotene, lutein, zeaxanthin, Kaempferol, and quercetin, which can play a promoting role in your body's defenses and skin health.

Ingredients:

- 1 cup Swiss chard
- 1 cup chopped Pineapple
- ½ cup cherries, pitted
- ½ cup blueberries
- 1 cup water

Instructions:

- ✓ Wash cherries and blueberries.
- ✓ Place all ingredients in a blender.
- ✓ Blend together while adding water until the desired consistency is reached.

32.   VITATURNIP

Thanks to the large amount of Vitamin A found in turnip greens, they are really good for your skin and hair health. They also have high amounts of vitamin C to help with building and repairing of collagen tissue in our skin.

Ingredients:

- 1 cup Turnip greens
- 1 Cucumber, sliced
- 1 cup Pomegranate juice
- ½ tsp ginger

Instructions:

- ✓ Wash turnip greens and cucumber.
- ✓ Place all ingredients in a blender.
- ✓ Blend together while adding water until the desired consistency is reached.

33.   NATURAL POWER

Almonds can help maintain your skin health. They're a great source of Vitamin E and other antioxidants that help in nourishing your skin. In some research, there are even indications that eating almonds can help our bodies fight skin cancer and reverse oxidative damages.

Ingredients:

- 8 almonds
- 1 cup blueberries
- 1 cup Strawberries
- 1 cup Greek Yoghurt
- ¼ tsp fresh Mint

Instructions:

- ✓ Wash the blueberries and strawberries.
- ✓ Place all ingredients in a blender.
- ✓ Blend together while adding water until the desired consistency is reached.

34.   D-TOX

Pistachios are a fabulous nut to include in our juices and meals. They contain a high amount of lutein and zeaxanthin, which have shown to improve your health and decrease the risk of cancer, particularly skin and eye diseases.

Ingredients:

- ½ cup pistachios, shelled
- 1 Carrot
- 1 Cucumber
- 1 cup Grapes
- 1 cup water

Instructions:

- ✓ Wash the carrot, cucumber and grapes.
- ✓ Place all ingredients in a blender.
- ✓ Blend together while adding water until the desired consistency is reached.

35.   OLYMJUS

Cacao powder is the original source of most chocolates we eat every day. Cacao powder is the best way to get all of the benefits from chocolate, as it contains a higher quantity of phytonutrients. Chocolate even has more antioxidants than tea, so it's better at reducing the risk of developing cancer.

Ingredients:

- 2 tbsp Cacao powder
- ½ Avocado, pitted, peeled
- 1 cup raspberries
- 1 cup Water
- 5 Almonds

Instructions:

- ✓ Place all ingredients in a blender.
- ✓ Blend together while adding water until the desired consistency is reached.

36.   CAROTEN-AID

Sunflower seeds are a perfect snack for your health. They help prevent cancer due to their high antioxidant content and they are a great source of selenium, a compound which has been found to have anti-cancer effects such as stimulating cancer cell apoptosis.

Ingredients:

- 2 tbsp Sunflower seeds
- ½ cup Pumpkin puree
- 1 cup apricot, sliced
- ½ tsp turmeric
- 1 cup water

Instructions:

- ✓ Place all ingredients in a blender.
- ✓ Blend together while adding water until the desired consistency is reached.

37.   VITAGOJILIN

Goji berries supply us with high levels of antioxidants, vitamin C, and vitamin A. All these nutrients are key in helping our immune system stay strong and prevent illnesses, ranging from a common cold to a chronic, dangerous disease like cancer. Goji berries promote healthy skin and act like a natural preventive measure against skin cancer.

Ingredients:

- 1 cup Goji Berries
- 1 cup Grapes
- 1 cup Coconut water
- 1 tbsp Flaxseed

Instructions:

- ✓ Wash grapes and goji berries.
- ✓ Place all ingredients in a blender.
- ✓ Blend together while adding water until the desired consistency is reached.

38. GRAPE GOODIE

Grapes are full of nutrients and vitamins, and phytonutrients like resveratrol that has been linked to anti-cancer effects on a variety of cancers. Grapes also provide us with beta-carotene, flavonoids, and antioxidants, which means that grapes are an incredible cancer-fighting food.

Ingredients:

- 1 cup grapes, seedless
- 1 banana
- 1 cup Cherries, pitted
- 1 cup Pomegranate juice

Instructions:

- ✓ Wash grapes and cherries.
- ✓ Place all ingredients in a blender.
- ✓ Blend together while adding water until the desired consistency is reached.

39.   GREENS'N'BERRIES

Blackberries are ranked among the highest antioxidant foods. This tells us that eating more Blackberries -and most berries in general- can help your system eliminate free radicals and prevent the proliferation of carcinogenic cells.

Ingredients:

- 1 cup Blackberries
- 1 cup Strawberries
- 1 cup Broccoli florets
- 1 tsp honey
- 1 cup water

Instructions:

- ✓ Wash the blackberries, strawberries and broccoli florets.
- ✓ Place all ingredients in a blender.
- ✓ Blend together while adding water until the desired consistency is reached.

40.   FIGFIGHTER

Figs and fig leaves are natural cancer-fighting foods. Figs contain powerful antioxidants, which have shown to be very effective to combat various types of cancer. More specifically, fig leaves can help prevent skin cancer due to its natural free radical damage fighters.

Ingredients:

- 2 Figs
- ¼ cup Fig leaves
- 1 cup chopped Papaya
- 1 cup chopped Mango, peeled and pitted
- 1 cup Greek yogurt

Instructions:

- ✓ Wash mango and fig leaves.
- ✓ Place all ingredients in a blender.
- ✓ Blend together while adding water until the desired consistency is reached.

41.   CITRUS INFUSION

Pomegranates are a good source of chemopreventive compounds, thanks to their polyphenols and lignans. These compounds are capable of inhibiting cancer cell proliferation and promote apoptosis.

Ingredients:

- 1 cup Pomegranate juice
- 2 grapefruits
- 1 cup diced Pineapple
- 1 tsp honey

Instructions:

- ✓ Wash the grapefruits and squeeze juice.
- ✓ Place all ingredients in a blender.
- ✓ Blend together while adding water until the desired consistency is reached.

42.   GREENIE

Matcha is the end-product of ground and processed green tea, but this powder has about 10 times the amount of antioxidants compared to green tea. Many studies have demonstrated the incredible effectiveness of matcha to prevent cancers of all sorts.

Ingredients:

- 1 tsp Matcha
- 1 Avocado, pitted, peeled
- ½ cup cherries, pitted
- 1 Celery stalk
- 1 cup water

Instructions:

- ✓ Wash the cherries and celery stalk.
- ✓ Place all ingredients in a blender.
- ✓ Blend together while adding water until the desired consistency is reached.

43.   O'FIG'IN

In this juice we are obtaining the properties of blueberries, almonds, figs and watermelon. All of these ingredients are well-known for their anti-cancer effects due to their high levels of vitamins and nutrients. With this powerful juice you can nourish your body and protect your skin.

Ingredients

- 1 cup Blueberries
- 1 Fig
- 1 cup chopped watermelon
- 5 almonds
- 1 cup water

Instructions:

- ✓ Wash the blueberries.
- ✓ Place all ingredients in a blender.
- ✓ Blend together while adding water until the desired consistency is reached.

44. SUNNY CHERRY JUICE

Sunny cherry juice is not only a tasty and wonderful juice but also an incredible source of vitamins and nutrients with many chemopreventive properties. We can see from the main ingredient – cherries - we obtain the flavonoids that give them their intense red coloration and possess these compounds with antioxidant, anti-inflammatory and cancer-preventing properties.

Ingredients:

- 2 cups cherries
- 1 cup diced Mango
- 1 cup chopped pineapple
- 1 cup Pomegranate juice

Instructions:

- ✓ Wash the cherries, mango and pineapple.
- ✓ Place all ingredients in a blender.
- ✓ Blend together while adding water until the desired consistency is reached.

45.   RISE'N'SHINE

Levels in blood of Vitamin D can be highly related to chances to get skin cancer. An important source of Vitamin D for our bodies is actually the sun, but extended exposure to the sun can negatively affect your skin. For this reason, we bring you the Rise'n'Shine juice that provides vitamin D from another source such as fortified Almond Milk.

Ingredients:

- 1 cup vitamin D fortified Almond milk
- 1 Banana, peeled
- 2 tbsp Flaxseed
- 4 almonds

Instructions:

- ✓ Place all ingredients in a blender.
- ✓ Blend together while adding water until the desired consistency is reached.

46. WAKE ME UP

Chia seeds have grown to be a very popular ingredient in health snacks as research has proven that chia seeds supply a very high amount of antioxidants so they can help speed up the skin's repair and prevent further damages, such as skin cancer.

Ingredients:

- 2 tbsp Chia seeds
- 1 banana, peeled
- 1 cup chopped Pineapple
- 1 tsp honey
- 1 cup water

Instructions:

- ✓ Place all ingredients in a blender.
- ✓ Blend together while adding water until the desired consistency is reached.

47.   CHOCOPOW

This juice will bring a lot of vitamin and nutrients, including the omega-3 fatty acids from the walnuts, the phytonutrients from cherries, the antioxidants from Cacao powder and many Vitamins com the almond milk; all of these in a delicious juice.

Ingredients:

- 4 Walnuts
- 1 cup cherries, pitted
- 1 tbsp Cacao powder
- 1 cup Almond milk

Instructions:

✓ Wash the cherries.

✓ Place all ingredients in a blender.

✓ Blend together while adding water until the desired consistency is reached.

48.   OXIJUICE

Tamarillo, or tree tomato, is an exotic and incredibly healthy fruit with high levels of vitamins and nutrients. With your aim to protect your skin and prevent skin cancer, this juice has to become part of your usual drinks.

Ingredients:

- 2 tamarillo, peeled
- 1 cup Green tea
- 1 cup strawberries

Instructions:

✓ Wash the tamarillo and strawberries.

✓ Place all ingredients in a blender.

✓ Blend together while adding water until the desired consistency is reached.

49.   MANGOODISH

Mangos are full of vitamins and beta-carotene. These compounds give mangos their anti-aging attributes, combined with their high levels of vitamins A and C, mangos even help to build collagen, repair skin damages, and prevent skin cancer.

Ingredients:

- 1 cup chopped mango
- 1 cup green tea
- ½ cup blueberries
- 1 tsp turmeric

Instructions:

- ✓ Wash the blueberries.
- ✓ Place all ingredients in a blender.
- ✓ Blend together while adding water until the desired consistency is reached.

MEALS

1.   Radish Hero

Description:

Radishes contain Vitamin C and antioxidants, which makes them quite effective in preventing skin diseases and inflammation. Adding radishes to your regular diet will make your skin more radiant and healthier. Steamed radishes have a very tender and delicious taste.

Ingredients:

- 20 radishes
- 2 tbsp water
- 1 tbsp olive oil
- salt and pepper to taste

How to prepare:

Wash radishes and trim the ends off of the radishes. Peel off a band of radish-skin from around the middle of the radish.

Add the radishes and the water and olive oil into a medium container.

Steam the radishes in a covered microwave safe container for 8 minutes, or until fork tender, and serve.

Nutritional facts:

Calories:109 Fat:10g, Carbohydrate:2g, Protein:1g

2. Asparagus the Great

Description:

Asparagus is an excellent source of anti-oxidants and it also contains a group of substances collectively called the saponins, known for their anti-inflammatory effect. Research has shown that these two kinds of compounds work together to reduce stress in the body. Reducing stress provides a healthier environment for preventing cancer.

Ingredients:

- 1 pound of asparagus
- 1 tablespoon olive oil
- Sea salt and pepper to taste

How to prepare:

Trim and wash asparagus. Trimming is easily accomplished by snapping the ends off where it snaps naturally.

Pour olive oil over asparagus and toss to coat.

Season generously with salt and pepper.

Place on a hot grill for 5 to 10 minutes for asparagus to become tender and remember to turn them often.

Nutritional facts:

Calories: 112 Fat: 6g Carbohydrates: 14g Protein: 3g

3.   Mount Chestnut's Soup

Description:

Research has shown that sweet chestnut offers antioxidant properties. One study examined sweet chestnut's ability to inhibit free radicals and found that its antioxidant potential was at least on a par with that of quercetin and Vitamin E

Ingredients:

- 3 tablespoon olive oil
- 1 medium carrot, finely chopped
- 1 celery rib, finely chopped
- 1/2 medium onion, finely chopped
- 2 cups cooked chestnuts
- 1 cup ruby port
- 1 thyme sprig
- 3 cups chicken stock or low-sodium broth
- 1/2 cup heavy cream
- Salt and freshly ground pepper

How to prepare:

Add the carrot, celery and onion and cook over moderately low heat, stirring, until softened, about 10 minutes.

Add the chestnuts and cook for 4 minutes.

Add the port and thyme and cook over moderately high heat until the port is reduced by half, about 4 minutes.

Add the stock and bring to a boil. Cover partially and simmer over low heat for 30 minutes.

Discard the thyme sprig. Add the cream to the soup. Working in batches, puree the soup in a blender.

Pour the soup back in the saucepan and bring to a simmer.

Season with salt and pepper and serve.

Nutritional facts:

Calories 325, Carbohydrates 10g, Protein 7g, Fat: 28g

4.   Celery Potatoe Salad

Description:

Celery is a great cancer-preventing food thanks to the bioflavonoid apigenin it contains. Adding this valuable vegetable to an earthy potato salad is going to be both tasty and nutritious. This salad may be served even a couple days after prepared, simply keep refrigerated and bring to room temperature when ready to eat.

Ingredients:

- 4 cups potatoes, peeled and sliced 1/4 inch thick
- 2 cups celery, chopped
- ½ cup onion, minced
- 2 tbsp lemon juice
- 1 tbsp mustard
- ½ cup flat leaf parsley, chopped

How to prepare:

Wash and place the potatoes in large boiling pot.

Cook the potatoes until they are tender but still retain their shape. Drain the stock and wait till potatoes are room temperature.

Toss with the potatoes, the chopped celery and parsley, and onions.

Whisk together the lemon juice and mustard and pour on the potatoes.

Season to taste with salt and pepper.

Nutritional facts:

Calories: 325 Cholesterol: 28 mg, Sodium 35 mg, Carbohydrates: 34 g, Protein 12g

5.   Cheesy Broccoli Soup

Description:

Broccoli is a great source of cancer-fighting compounds. To maximize the benefits of broccoli, avoid overcooking it and better eat it raw or slightly steamed. Eating raw, slightly crushed broccoli will result in far better absortion of the key components found in this vegetable, as cooking broccoli will reduce in large amount the availability of sulforaphane — the key cancer fighting chemical compound in broccoli.

Ingredients:

- 3 tbsp potato starch
- 3 tbsp olive oil
- 1 small sweet onion, diced
- 2 stalks of celery diced
- pepper to taste
- 6 cups chicken stock
- 4 cups chopped broccoli
- 2 cups whole organic milk or almond milk
- 3 cups shredded cheddar cheese
- ½ tsp nutmeg

How to prepare:

In a stock pot, sauté onions and celery until tender (about 5 minutes).

Add in potato starch and stir.

Add chicken stock to stock pot slowly while stirring.

Slowly add the chopped broccoli and simmer over low heat for 30 minutes.

Stir in milk and cheese and allow to heat through (about 5 more minutes).

Serve with some shredded cheddar cheese.

Nutritional facts:

Calories: 252 Fat: 15g Carbohydrates: 12g Protein: 10g

6.   Epic Banana Bread

Description:

This bread is perfect for breakfast or for snacking. Banana is great not just for skin, but one's overall health as well. There are many powerful nutrients contained in this fruit that make it the perfect addition to your daily meals.

Ingredients:

- 6 organic eggs
- 2 ripe organic bananas, mashed
- 1 tbsp raw honey
- ⅓ cup melted coconut oil (cooled)
- ½ tsp unrefined sea salt
- ½ cup coconut flour
- ½ tsp baking soda
- 1 cup chopped raw pecans or walnuts

How to prepare:

Preheat oven to 350 F.

In a large bowl combine eggs, honey, and the cooled coconut oil and mix well.

In a small bowl combine coconut flour, salt, baking soda and stir well.

Add the contents of the small bowl to the large bowl and stir until there are no more lumps.

Add in bananas and mix until well blended.

Pour batter into 2 greased mini bread pans or 1 5"x9" loaf pan.

Bake for 40-50 minutes or until lightly browned

Nutritional facts:

Calories: 162 Fat: 11g Carbohydrates: 10g Protein: 5g

7. Carotene Carrot Cake

Description:

Carrots are also an important vegetable to include in your diet if you are worried about developing skin cancer. Because of their high beta-carotene content, carrots are great at protecting the skin against harmful ultraviolet radiation from the sun. Transform carrots into a cupcake and even kids will love it.

Ingredients:

- ¼ cup whole wheat flour
- ¼ tsp salt
- 1 tsp cinnamon
- 3 large eggs
- ¼ cup olive oil
- ½ cup raw unfiltered honey
- 1 tbsp vanilla extract
- 1 cup grated carrots
- chopped walnuts and raisins (½ cup chopped and some to sprinkle on top of frosting.)

Cream Cheese Icing:

- 16 oz pkg. softened organic cream cheese

- 2 tsp vanilla extract

- 2 tbsp of raw unfiltered honey

How to prepare:

Preheat oven to 350º F.

Combine the ingredients and put in an olive oil spread pan. Bake for 16-30 minutes. Insert a Knife or fork and when it comes out clean you will know it is ready.

For the frosting combine the organic cream cheese, vanilla, honey, and salt with 4 tbsp of water. Whip on high speed for 4 minutes.

This will create a silky smooth frosting. Spread over the cake or cupcakes to create your carrot cake cupcake.

Nutritional facts:

Calories: 157 Fat: 11g Carbs: 16g Protein: 4g

8.   Sorrel Salad Delight

Description:

Sorrel can strengthen eyesight, improve digestion, build stronger bones, increase circulation, prevent cancer, minimize specific skin problems, lower blood pressure, and slow down aging. Sorrel is an impressive herb that is used in many countries around the world. Although it is mainly cultivated due to its sharp, tangy taste, sorrel also has a wide range of health benefits linked with it.

Ingredients:

- ½ cup greek yogurt
- 1 tbsp olive oil
- 1 tbsp lime juice
- 1 tbsp minced chives
- 1 tsp honey
- 1½ avocado
- ¼ tsp mustard
- ½ cup sorrel
- ½ cup hearts of romaine
- ¼ cup endive leaves

- ¼ cup parsley

- 2 tbsp Basil leaves

How to prepare:

Mix all dressing ingredients together in a bowl.

Mix all salad ingredients in a larger bowl.

Slice avocado in small squares and mix into salad.

Nutritional facts:

Calories: 212, Carbohydrates 16g, Protein 8g

9.   Roasted Happy Seeds

Description:

A quick snack available for anyone, especially for our kids. Easy to prepare and lasts for a long time. Vitamin E is an important nutrient for a healthy skin and you can find this anti-oxidant in pistachios. Vitamin E helps the body protect the skin from damaging UV rays, and also plays a role in preventing skin disease and making our skin vigorous and more appealing.

Ingredients:

- 2 cups shelled pistachios

How to prepare:

Preheat oven to 350 degrees F.

Spread the pistachios evenly on a rimmed cookie sheet. Bake for 6 to 8 minutes and you will notice their pleasant smell in the air.

Remove from oven and transfer to a plate immediately.

Let the pistachios cool and then you can store them.

They taste amazing in baking recipes when they are toasted.

Nutritional facts:

Serving Size for ½ cup: Calories: 165, Fat: 14 g, Carbs: 11g, Protein: 7g

10.   Futuristic Veggie Chips

Description:

Oven-fried zucchini chips taste like they're fried, yet they are baked and amazingly crispy. These chips make a healthy substitute for French fries. Zucchini is rich in Vitamins A and C as well as antioxidants which can benefit your skin in many ways. Regular consumption of zucchini helps restore the moisture of your skin, providing you with a glowing skin.

Ingredients:

- 3 small zucchini, sliced into ¼- inch rounds
- 2 tbsp olive oil
- ½ cup seasoned bread crumbs
- 2 tbsp grated Parmesan cheese
- 2 tsp fresh oregano

How to prepare:

Preheat oven to 350 degrees F (175 degrees C).

Place zucchini in a bowl. Drizzle olive oil over zucchini and stir to coat; add bread crumbs and toss to coat.

Spread coated zucchini onto a flat baking sheet.

Sprinkle Parmesan cheese and oregano over coated zucchini.

Bake in the preheated oven until zucchini are tender and cheese is browned (about 15 minutes).

Nutritional facts:

1 Serving (10 chips) Calories:94, Total fat: 2g, Carbohydrates: 10g, Protein: 5g, Sodium 323mg

11.   BlueBerry Almond Yogurt

Description:

The health benefits of yogurt have always been important to mankind. Yogurt is a great source of many vitamins and minerals that are also present in milk. Also, yogurt provides a good source of probiotics and easily digestible proteins. Combine this with the antioxidants in blueberries and the healthy oils in almonds, and you will have a powerful snack to prevent skin cancer.

Ingredients:

- 1 cup organic blueberries
- 2 cups organic plain yogurt with live active yogurt cultures or probiotics
- ½ cup chopped almonds

How to prepare:

Place 2 cups of organic yogurt in a medium to large bowl

Add 1 cup organic blueberries to the bowl and lightly mix with the yogurt

Pour the chopped almonds into the bowl and mix lightly

Serve into small cups; makes for 3 servings.

Refrigerate your yogurt until ready to eat.

Nutritional facts (per serving of one small cup):

Calories: 348 Fat: 20g Carbohydrates: 31g Protein: 14g

12.   Roasted Organic Kohlrabi & Sweet Potato

Description:

Sweet potatoes, one of the oldest vegetables known to man, are one of the most nutritious vegetables and contain plenty of nutrients with skin cancer fighting properties. Kohlrabi is a good source of vitamin-C and presents a mild taste similar to broccoli. Vitamin C (ascorbic acid) is a water-soluble vitamin, and powerful anti-oxidant that helps remove harmful free-radicals from all over the body.

Ingredients:

- 1 cup cubed sweet potatoes (skin removed)
- 1 cup cubed kohlrabi (skin removed)
- 1 tbsp olive oil
- 5 sprigs of fresh thyme
- salt and pepper to taste

How to prepare:

Mix all ingredients together and roast in a 450 F oven for 25 minutes, turning half way through the cooking time.

Nutritional facts:

Size 1 cup, calories 156, carbs 16g, fat 10g, protein 2g

13.   Fresh Summer Organic Salsa

Description:

Avocados are brimming with nutrients that reduce the risk of skin cancer. Avocados top the list of the best dietary sources of glutathione, an important antioxidant.

Ingredients:

- 1 tbsp lime juice
- ½ cup cilantro chopped
- 2 tbsp organic olive oil
- ¼ tsp sea salt
- ¼ tsp pepper
- 2 cups organic corn
- 3 avocados sliced into smaller pieces
- 2 and ½ cups diced tomatoes
- ¼ cup red onion diced very well

How to prepare:

In a large bowl, stir the cilantro, olive oil, lime juice, salt and pepper.

Combine with the cherry tomatoes, avocado, red onion and corn.

Stir gently and serve at room temperature.

Nutritional facts:

Calories: 203, Fat 16g, Carbohydrates 17g, Protein 4g

14.   Organic Guacamole

Description:

Avocados are the primary ingredient in guacamole, a popular and healthy food commonly used as a spread or dip. Being a great source of essential oils, vitamins, and the antioxidant glutathione, avocados are an excellent choice as a healthy snack to prevent skin cancer.

Ingredients:

- 2 avocados halved, pitted, and removed from peel
- ½ tsp salt
- ¼ tsp pepper
- ¼ cup fresh tomatoes, diced up
- ½ of a lime, juice squeezed out (about 1 tbsp)
- 2 tbsp fresh cilantro, chopped
- 1 tbsp red onion (optional)

How to prepare:

Combine all ingredients and mash with fork.

Serve immediately.

Nutritional facts:

Calories: 142 Fat: 12g Carbohydrates: 8g Protein: 4g

15.   Organic Fruit Splash

Description:

Strawberries are super fruits, bursting with powerful anti-oxidants and loads of vitamin C that will provide your skin with nourishing nutrients for healthy happy skin. Avocados are brimming with nutrients that can reduce the risk of skin cancer. Make together into a salad and your skin will benefit!

Ingredients: (4 servings)

- 2 avocados peeled and pitted
- 1 cup strawberries finely chopped
- 2 tbsp chopped cilantro
- 1 tbsp organic olive oil
- ¼ tsp unrefined sea salt

How to prepare:

Slice the peeled and pitted avocadoes into bitesize cubes.

Place the avocado cubes in a large bowl.

Add the remaining ingredients to the large bowl and mix.

Nutritional facts:

Calories: 264, Fat: 19g, Carbs: 18g, Protein: 6g

16. Veggie Noodles

Description:

Craving Thai Food, but need a Raw, Vegan alternative? This veggie noodle recipe is almost easier than calling for take-out. It'll make your head spin it's so fast and delicious. This meal would provide an excellent source of vitamins and nutrients well-recognized in preventing skin cancer.

Ingredients:

- 2 zucchini
- 1 carrot
- 2 green onions
- ½ cup mushrooms
- ½ cup cauliflower
- ½ cup mung bean sprouts
- 2 tbsp sesame oil
- 1 tbsp lemon juice
- 1 tsp garlic

How to prepare:

Use a spiralizer (or mandoline, or peeler) to create your noodles. Add in veggies of your choice then top with the sauce. It tastes even better after it sits for a day to soak the flavors.

Nutritional facts:

Serving Size: 356: Calories: 185, Total Fat: 15g, Carbs: 31g, Protein 8g

17.   Popeyes' Secret

Description:

When it comes to the best foods for preventing skin cancer, it is difficult to beat the superfood kale. This relatively unknown member of the cabbage family is a superhero vegetable cram-full of skin cancer preventing nutrients, including vitamin C and beta-carotene (kale contains more than 5 times the beta-carotene of broccoli). As a result of its high content of vitamin C and beta-carotene as well as a number of other antioxidant phytonutrients, kale is at the top of the list of vegetables with the highest ORAC rating. ORAC, or Oxygen Radical Absorbance Capacity, is a measure of the total antioxidant power of foods. Kale can be eaten raw, for example in salads. The hearty green leaves of kale can also be transformed into a savory side dish by sautéing them and adding onions, garlic and a drizzle of olive oil.

Ingredients:

- 1 cup uncooked quinoa (rinsed)

- 2 tbsp olive oil

- 1 large clove of garlic (minced)

- 1 cup fresh spinach

- 2 cups fresh kale
- 2-3 tsp lemon juice (start with 2 tsp, and if you would like more add another tsp)
- 2 tbsp raw sunflower seeds or raw pecans (chopped in small pieces)
- ⅓ cup raw shredded parmesan cheese

How to prepare:

Rinse your dried quinoa several times

Boil your quinoa in salted water and cook for 20 minutes.

Drain and rinse in cold water, set aside.

In a large skillet add olive oil and garlic.

Toss your garlic for about a minute and then add your kale and spinach.

Cook several minutes to wilt your spinach and kale.

Add your quinoa, lemon juice and parmesan cheese.

Cook for 2 minutes.

Toss in your raw sunflower seeds or raw pecans and cook another minute.

Serve hot or cold.

Nutritional facts:

Calories: 212, Fat: 12 g Carbs: 18g, Protein: 6g

18.   Sunset Chips

Description:

Garlic offers a number of health benefits due to the allicin it contains. Allicin has natural benefits in fighting aging, infections, and preventing skin cancer

Ingredients:

- 2 sweet potatoes of choice (sweet, russet, or red)
- 1 tbsp coconut oil or olive oil
- 3 sprigs of fresh rosemary
- 2 cloves minced garlic
- sea salt to taste

How to prepare:

Preheat oven to 400ºF.

Finely slice the potatoes

Place potato slices in a bowl and drizzle with coconut oil or olive oil (or both) and mince the garlic and season with sea salt.

Add the sprigs of rosemary and toss until well coated.

Set on a flat oven pan and bake for roughly 20 minutes or until golden brown and crisp.

Allow to fully cool and then serve. You can also store in a cool dry place inside a bag.

Nutritional facts:

Calories: 144 Fat: 10 g Protein: 3 g

19.   Crunchy Coconut Chips

Description:

Coconut oil has a rich content of healthy fats that our body needs to nourish our tissues, including our skin. By eating this healthy fats regularly, we will be preventing skin cancer and noticing better health all-around.

Ingredients:

- ½ cup organic extra virgin coconut oil

- 3 cups organic coconut flakes

- ½ tsp sea salt (more if you want extra salty)

How to prepare:

Preheat oven to 300 degrees

Place the coconut flakes in a large bowl and mix with the coconut oil and salt to taste.

Place the coconut-coated flakes on a flat baking pan.

Bake a total of 8 minutes, until golden brown. Watch carefully, it browns quickly.

Allow to cool, and then pour onto a party bowl – enjoy!

Nutritional facts:

Calories: 210, Fat: 8g, Protein 1g, Carbs 3g

20.   Organic Potato Boats

Description:

Apart from being used as a delicious food source, potatoes have an important role to play in skincare as well. As mentioned before, they are rich in vitamin C which is vital for maintaining a healthy skin.

Ingredients:

- Skins of 3 potatoes, organic, cooked
- 8 cooked baconstrips, chopped
- 1 cup shredded cheese of your preference
- salt and pepper to taste
- 1 avocado, peeled, pitted, and cubed
- ½ cup sour cream

How to prepare:

In a small bowl, mix the avocado cubes, chopped cooked bacon, and shredded cheese.

Preheat oven to 400F.

Cut the potatoe skins in half to make boatshaped.

Take your potato skin boats with empty side up and lay on a flat baking pan.

Fill the potato boats with the avocado mix from the small bowl.

Cover with shredded cheese of your preference.

Bake for 8 minutes or until shredded cheese begins to appear tannish-brown.

Remove from oven and allow to cool.

Top your potatoe boats with sour cream, salt and pepper and serve.

Nutritional facts:

Calories: 210, Fat: 17g, Protein 6g, Carbs 26g

21. Garlic's Treaty

Description:

Garlic has a lot of medicinal properties for skin. Having natural healing properties, garlic helps our skin stay strong and young, as well to heal. Garlic is a powerful antioxidant, so it can act as an important preventing-agent against skin cancer.

Ingredients:

- 7 large cubed pieces of bread of choice (If gluten free, use gluten free bread)
- 3 tbsp olive oil
- ½ tsp unrefined garlic salt
- ½ tsp Italian seasoning
- 2 tbsp grated parmesan cheese

How to prepare:

Preheat oven to 300 F.

If using fresh bread, cut the bread into cubes.

Place bread cubes into a bowl.

Mix the olive oil, salt and seasoning in a small bowl, then pour over the bread cubes and toss well so that the bread cubes get evenly coated.

Sprinkle with parmesan cheese and toss bread cubes until they are all evenly coated.

Set on a flat baking sheet and bake for 25 minutes, turning them over at the 15 minute mark.

Allow to cool and store in an air tight container.

Nutritional facts:

Calories: 68, Fat: 3g, Protein 2g, Carbs 8g

22. Pumpkinny Cheesecake

Description:

Beta-carotene (a carotenoid better known as vitamin A), found in the bright orange pulp of pumpkins is known to protect skin cells from oxidative damage caused by free radicals. It is also well known due to its potential anti-cancer, anti-aging and immune-enhancing effects. Pumpkin is also a good source of vitamin C; another powerful antioxidant that combats free radicals and prevents skin cancer.

Ingredients:

Crust:

- 1 cup of nuts of your choice (I used raw walnuts and almonds)
- 4-5 dates
- Dash of sea salt

Filling:

- 16 oz of cream cheese (at room temperature)
- 1 cup of ricotta cheese
- ¼ cup sour cream

- 2 cups of pumpkin puree

- 3 eggs plus 1 egg yolk

- ¾ cup of organic honey

- ½ tsp ground cinnamon

- ¼ tsp nutmeg

- ¼ tsp ground cloves

- 2 tbsp oat flour

- 1 tsp vanilla extract

Whipping cream

- 1 pint of whole cream

- Honey to taste

How to prepare:

To make crust:

Grind all crust ingredients in a food processor until crumbly and somewhat sticky.

To prepare pumpkin puree:

Cut each pumpkin in half, scoop out seeds, and place on a parchment lined cooking sheet, Bake at 350 degrees for 45 minutes.

Allow to cool, scoop out pumpkin and put in a food

processor until pureed to consistency.

To make filling:

Beat cream cheese until smooth.

Add pumpkin and sour cream, and add oat flour and vanilla.

Add eggs, egg yolk, ricotta, honey and spices, then mix.

Beat together until well mixed.

Pour on top of crust in springform pan, spreading out evenly.

Bake at 350 degrees for 45 minutes to 1 hour.

Allow to cool, cover with plastic and chill for 2 hours.

To make whipping cream:

Whip whole cream in a chilled bowl, add honey to sweeten taste

To complete Pumpkinny Cheesecake:

Top cheesecake with whipped cream. Sprinkle with fresh ground nutmeg.

The key with using a springform pan is to grease well the pan and side-edges with a butter knife before "springing" it.

Nutritional facts:

Calories: 275, Fat: 25g, Carbs: 29g, Protein: 5g

23.   Wild Garlic Salmon

Description:

New research suggests that twice-weekly consumption of salmon could protect against skin cancer. The high levels of omega-3 fat found in this oily fish are also great for overall skin health. Salmon reduces inflammation as opposed to redmeats, which increase inflammation.

Ingredients:

- 1 tbsp olive oil
- 1 clove garlic, minced
- ¼ tsp garlic salt
- ¼ tsp ground black pepper
- 1 pound wild-caught salmon

How to prepare:

In a small bowl, mix the minced garlic, olive oil, garlic salt, and pepper.

Cut the salmon into serving-size filets..

Rest the salmon filets on a glass baking dish.

Coat the salmon filets with the mix from the small bowl.

Preheat oven to 400 degrees F (200 degrees C).

Place the baking dish in the preheated oven, and bake salmon uncovered for 20 minutes (until easily flaked with a fork).

Nutritional facts:

Calories: 32, Carbs 14g, Fat 21g, Protein 18g

24.   Root Juice

Description:

Beetroot is rich in betacyanin, a powerful anticancer agent. Also, beetroot will help your skin stay healthy thanks to the many minerals and vitamins it provides.

Ingredients:

- 1 raw beetroot
- 2 carrots
- 10 radishes
- ½ lemon
- 2 apples

How to prepare:

Peel the lemon to remove the outer skin.

Wash the vegetables and chop them into chunks.

Core the apples and chop into about ten pieces.

Put everything into the juicer, then after juiced, chill the mixture before drinking.

Nutritional facts:

Calories 19, Carbs 5g, Protein 1g

25.   Fruity Salmon

Description:

A quick, healthy dinner option, as well as low-calorie. Wild-caught salmon is a super food because of its omega-3 fatty acid content so it is an essential recipe for adding more healthy oils to our cancer-preventing diet.

Ingredients:

- 1 Pound Wild-caught Salmon, cut into 4 filets
- 2 Oranges, thinly sliced
- ¾ cup Fresh Squeezed Orange Juice
- 1 tbsp Fresh Squeezed Lime Juice
- 2 tbsp olive oil or coconut oil
- 1 tbsp organic sugar or raw
- ½ tsp salt
- ¼ tsp Chipotle Pepper or Cayenne Pepper or Chili Powder
- Optional—1 small bunch of fresh Thyme sprigs as garnish
- Optional—fresh Lemon wedges for serving

How to prepare:

Preheat oven to 450ºF.

Slice two oranges into very thin slices, discard ends, and set aside.

Squeeze orange and lime with a citrus juicer.

Measure out ¼ cup fresh orange juice and 2 tablespoons fresh lime juice and add to a small glass bowl along with the lemon zest. Whisk in coconut oil or olive oil and sugar or honey, along with salt and pepper.

Line a baking sheet with parchment paper.

Using a basting brush, brush one side of each of the salmon filets with the citrus mixture then arrange filets on top of parchment paper. Brush tops of salmon with the citrus mixture.

Optional, wash sprigs of fresh thyme. Tear off a few of the bottom leaves of each sprig. Sprinkle on top of orange slices.

Bake 10 to 12 minutes or until salmon is cooked through.

Optional—top with fresh sprigs of thyme and serve with lemon wedges.

Nutritional facts:

Calories 275, Carbs 22g, Fat 19g, Protein 24g

26.   Painted Green Swiss Salad

Description:

The colorful additions of grapefruit and red oranges complement terrificly with the nutritious beetroot and swiss cheese in this tasty salad filled with anti-oxidants to prevent skin cancer.

Ingredients:

For the salad:

- 6 oz spring green mix, spinash, or baby kale

- 200g swiss cheese, grated

- 240g beetroot

- 1 ripe grapefruit

- 1 ripe blood orange

- 180g walnuts

For the dressing:

- 3 tbsp olive oil

- 1 tbsp red wine vinegar

- 2 tsp mustard

- Salt, pinch

How to prepare:

Wash and place in salad bowl the spring greens (or spinach or kale).

Chop the walnuts and beetroot into small pieces.

Section the grapefruit and orange, removing the fruit in small bitesize chunks.

Mix the nuts, beetroot, grapefruit and orange with the spring greens (or spinach or kale).

Sprinkle the grated Swiss cheese on top of salad.

In a small bowl, combine the olive oil, vinegar, mustard, and pinch of salt to make the dressing.

Drizzle the dressing on the salad and serve.

Nutritional facts:

Calories 215, Carbs 12g, Fat 16g, Protein 9g

27.   Peelicious Honey Citrus

Description:

Researchers have found that d-limonene (the major components in orange peel) can reduce the occurrence of squamous cell carcinoma, which is a dangerous form of skin cancer. Study participants who regularly consume citrus fruit skin, significantly reduce skin cancer rate than just eating the inside of the fruit.

Ingredients:

- 5 lemon peels, cut into ½ inch strips
- 5 orange peels, cut into ½ inch strips
- 1 cup organic honey
- 1 cup water

How to prepare:

Boil the lemon and orange peels in water for 15 minutes.

Let peels cool, then drain the water and let rest.

Place a baking sheet on a flat pan and pour a thin layer of the honey across the entire surface.

Roll the lemon and orange strips on the honey pan and set aside in a serving bowl.

Nutritional facts:

Calories 75, Potassium 64mg, Carbs 18g, Fat 1g

28.   Healthy Beef's Gift

Description:

Grass-fed beef provides a healthier amount of omega fatty acids when compared to other kinds of beef, and also contains a solid serving of protein, which is helpful to keep skin with less wrinkles and looking healthier by giving our body what it needs to build elastic tissue and collagen.

Ingredients:

- 1 pound grass-fed beef, cut of your choice
- 3 sprigs oregano
- 3 sprigs parsley
- 2 cloves garlic
- 3 tbsp olive oil
- 1 teaspoon salt
- ¼ tsp pepper

How to prepare:

Blend together the olive oil, garlic cloves, thyme, parsley, oregano, and salt, then place in a bowl.

Rub the blended mix on meat, then let it marinate 2 hours at room temperature or overnight in the refrigerator, turning meat once or twice.

Heat a medium cast-iron pan over medium heat.

Sear meat on pan until it has a brown crust

Preheat oven to 400°F, and then transfer pan to oven and roast meat for 15-25 minutes, until desired degree of doneness is reached.

Remove pan from oven and let meat cool to desired serving temperature.

Nutritional facts:

Calories 183, fat 9g, carbs 16g, protein 18g

29.   Veggie-Stars

Description:

Beetroot is your everyday superfood. They are a nutritional dynamo and a great excellent example of how food can help keep us healthy. Beetroot's rich color derives from the pigment betacyanin which is a powerful cancer fighting compound. Beetroot also has high content of many vitamins and minerals, including phosphorous, iron, folic acid, and magnesium.

Ingredients:

- 250g cooked beetroot dipped in vinegar (not pickled)
- 10 oz beans of choice, drained & rinsed
- 2 garlic cloves, crushed
- 1 oz chives, minced
- 2 tbsp olive oil
- ¼ tsp salt
- ¼ tsp pepper

How to prepare:

Chop the beetroot into small dice, set aside in a medium bowl.

Blend together the chives, olive oil, salt, pepper, beans, and garlic.

Place the blended mix into the beetroot bowl and mix together.

Serve as a spread for wheat crackers or as a dip for celery and carrots.

Nutritional facts:

Calories 184, Carbs 6g, Fat 14g, Protein 5g

30.   Hale Kale Salad with Tomatoes

Description:

This is the basic recipe for a delicious and quick kale salad with tomatoes. You can of course add other ingredients. Kale contains very high content of lutein and zeaxanthin, which are natural chemicals that are able to neutralize the harmful free radicals created by exposure to sunlight.

Ingredients:

- 1 bunch kale leaves
- 1 medium or large avocado
- 2 tomatoes
- ½ cup lemon juice
- 2 tsp of salt
- Pinch of pepper

How to prepare:

To prepare the kale leaves: glide your thumbnail down the stem, separating the leaf from the stem. Rip the leaves into small pieces.

Cut the avocado in half lengthwise and remove the pit. Raise out each avocado half and place on the kale leaves.

Add the lemon juice, cayenne, and salt to taste.

Puree the avocado with the kale as to coat the kale with the creamy avocado mixture.

Cut the tomatoes in small slices and add them in the bowl.

Nutritional facts:

Calories 372, fat 32g, carbs 41g, protein 8g

31. Betterave French Soup

Description:

Beetroot is your everyday superfood. They are a nutritional dynamo and a great excellent example of how food can help keep us healthy. Beetroot's rich color derives from the pigment betacyanin which is a powerful cancer fighting compound. Beetroot also has high content of many vitamins and minerals, including phosphorous, iron, folic acid, and magnesium.

Ingredients:

- 3 tablespoons olive oil
- 1 onion, minced
- 2 cloves garlic, minced
- 5 beets, peeled and chopped
- 1 cup beef or chicken stock per choice
- ½ tsp salt and freshly ground pepper

How to prepare:

Warm olive oil in a large saucepan over medium heat. Stir in the minced garlic and onion until lightly brown.

Add the beats, salts and pepper, and cook for 2 minutes.

Stir in stock until it reaches a light boil and then cover. In 18-25 minutes, beets will be tender.

Remove from heat until it cool to room temperature.

In 1 cup portions, add soup to a blender and liquefy.

Return soup to saucepan, and gently heat through to desired serving temperature.

Nutritional facts:

Calories 32, Carbs 6g, Fat 1g, Protein 1g

32.   Premium Squash Noodles

Description:

Squash is an excellent source of Vitamin A. The so called 'noodles' will be tossed with feta cheese and vegetables. This is one of the easiest way to cook squash.

Ingredients:

- 1 spaghetti squash, halved and seeded

- 1 garlic clove, minced

- 2½ tbsp olive oil

- ½ onion, chopped

- 2 tbsp basil, minced

- 2 tbsp black olives, sliced

- 2 cups tomatoes, chopped

- ¾ cup crumbled feta cheese

How to prepare:

Preheat oven to 350 degrees F (170 degrees C).

Rest the spaghetti squash with cut side's face down on a baking sheet, and bake for 18 minutes in the preheated oven.

Take squash out of oven and let it cool.

Pour olive oil on a skillet over medium heat. Add the chopped onions, basil, garlic, tomatoes, and sliced olives. Stir until mix is cooked for 2 minutes.

Use a large spoon to scoop the squash and place in a large bowl.

Pour the skillet mix on top of the squash, toss in the crumbled feta cheese, and serve.

Nutritional facts:

Calories: 148, carbs 12g, Fat 9g, Protein 4g

33.   Anti-inflamatory Turmeric Tea

Description:

Turmeric is a deep orange root that is used as a spice in a lot of recipes due to its exotic flavor and impressive health benefits. Turmeric has shown to contain strong anti-oxidant activity, making it valuable in preventing cancer. Another tremendous benefit of turmeric is its potent anti-inflammatory activity, which can be a great tool to fight signs of aging.

Ingredients:

- 32 oz boiling water
- ½ tbsp turmeric powder
- 1 tbsp olive oil
- 1 tbsp ginger, minced
- 1 cup cilantro, chopped
- 1 garlic clove, peeled and crushed
- 1 lemon, juiced
- 2 tbsp organic honey

How to prepare:

Put water on the stove to boil.

Combine the olive oil, turmeric powder, ginger, cilantro, garlic, lemon juice, and honey in a teapot.

Pour boiling water into the teapot and let it soak for 15 minutes. Strain and serve.

Nutritional facts:

Calories 87, Carbs 17g, Fat 6g, Protein 5g

34.   Peanut Butter Yogurt Dip

Description:

A wonderfully balanced dip with organic yogurt, cinnamon, organic peanut butter, honey, and vanilla. It's delicious with apples, graham crackers, and bananas.

Ingredients:

- 1 cup organic whole plain yogurt
- 4 tbsp organic peanut butter
- 1 tsp vanilla extract
- 2 tsp organic honey
- 1 tsp cinnamon

How to prepare:

Mix all ingredients in a small bowl until uniform.

Serve with snack of choice.

Store remaining in a refrigerated ambient.

Nutritional facts:

Calories 65, fat 5g, carbs 6g, protein 3g

35. Avocado's Madness

Description:

Avocados are rich in cancer-fighting chemicals, which are most plentiful in the darker green portion of the avocado that's nearest to the peel.

Ingredients:

- 2 avocados - peeled, pitted and diced
- 1 lemon, juiced
- 2 mangos - peeled, seeded and diced
- 1 small red onion, chopped
- ¼ tsp salt
- ¼ tsp ground pepper
- 1 tbsp cilantro, chopped

How to prepare:

Place the diced avocado in a serving bowl, and mix with the lemon juice.

Add the mango dices, chopped onion, ground pepper, chopped cilantro and salt, then mix till uniform.

Nutritional facts:

Calories: 252, Carbs 34g, Fats: 15g, Protein: 6g

36.   Fresh Morning Salad

Description:

A simple spinach salad special by adding avocado, spices and fresh cilantro. Make it ahead, refrigerate and then toss right before serving.

Ingredients:

- 10 oz baby spinach
- 3 tbsp fresh lemon juice
- 3 tbsp olive oil
- ¼ cup cilantro, chopped
- 1 tsp organic sugar
- ¼ tsp ground cumin
- ¼ tsp salt
- Pinch of ground pepper
- 2 avocados, peeled, pitted and cubed
- ½ cup minced red onion

How to prepare:

Whisk lime juice, cumin, olive oil, sugar, cilantro, salt and pepper in a large serving bowl.

Toss in avocado and minced red onion.

Place baby spinach on top. (Salad can be prepared and refrigerated up to 2 hours ahead.) Mix spinach with the rest right before serving.

Nutritional facts:

Calories: 89, Fat 7g, Carbs 5g, protein 6g

37.   Green Beans Sticks

Description:

Rich in antioxidants and detoxifying nutrients, green beans contain fiber, antioxidants, amino acids, folic acid, vitamin A, and vitamin C, all of which are very useful in preventing skin cancer.

Ingredients:

- 12 oz green beans, ends trimmed
- 3 tbsp olive oil
- 2 garlic cloves, minced
- ½ tsp red pepper
- 1 tbsp lemon zest
- ¼ tsp salt
- ¼ tsp ground pepper

How to prepare:

Place green beans in a large stock pot of well salted boiling water for 2 to 4 minutes. You will notice they turn bright green and crispier.

Drain and shock in an empty bowl to allow to cool.

Heat a large heavy skillet over medium heat. Add the olive oil, garlic and red pepper.

Sauté until fragrant, for about 30 seconds.

Add the green beans and continue to sauté for about 5 minutes.

Add lemon zest and season with salt and pepper.

Nutritional facts:

Calories: 366, Fats: 8g, Protein: 6g, Carbs 16g

38.   Modern Cauliflower Slices

Description:

Add some color to your cauliflower with turmeric. These cauliflower steaks are easy to prepare and would make a delicious appetizer or main dish. Turmeric contains approximately 2% curcumin and is one of the most important component it has. Curcumin plays an important role in helping our skin heal from exposure to ultraviolet rays so it is a key player in preventing skin cancer.

Ingredients:

- 1 large cauliflower
- ½ cup olive oil
- 2 tsp ground turmeric
- Thinly sliced red chili, to serve
- Thinly sliced green pepper, to serve
- Thinly sliced yellow pepper, to serve

How to prepare:

Cut the cauliflower into several 2 cm thick slices, leaving base intact.

Place slices on a non-stick frying pan over medium-high heat for 2 to 3 minutes and turn each side or until golden.

Line 2 baking trays with foil.

Transfer slices to the foil-lined baking tray.

Whisk the ground turmeric with the olive oil in a small bowl. Brush over steaks.

Preheat oven to 360 F.

Roast cauliflower in the oven for 12-15 minutes or until tender and crisp.

Scatter with thinly sliced red chili, green pepper, and yellow pepper, and serve.

Nutritional facts:

Calories: 156, Carbs 14g, Fats: 4g, Protein: 5g

39.   Cheesy Asparagus Saves the Day

Description:

Asparagus is a very good source of fiber, folic acid, vitamin C, and vitamin A, so adding asparagus to our regular die twill be smart, healthy decision.

Ingredients:

- 1 bunch asparagus (about 3/4 pound), ends trimmed
- 1 garlic clove, minced
- 1 tbsp olive oil
- ¼ cup parmesan cheese, grated finely
- ¼ cup chopped walnuts
- ¼ cup fresh thyme leaves
- ¼ tsp salt
- ¼ tsp ground pepper

How to prepare:

Place the asparagus in boiling water and cook for about 3 minutes until fragrant.

Stir in the boiling asparagus the thyme leaves and minced garlic, and cook for an additional 1 minute.

Remove from heat, toss in the cheese and mix.

Season with salt and pepper.

Add the chopped walnuts over the warm cheesed asparagus, and serve.

Nutritional facts:

134 calories; carbs 6g, fat 4g; protein 4 g

40.   Shrimps gone Wild

Description:

Shrimp are supercharged with vitamin B12 and selenium. Shrimp also provide a good source of astaxanthin, an antioxidant that can help our bodies prevent skin cancer. In addition, shrimp provide good amounts of vitamin A, magnesium, phosphorous, and zinc.

Ingredients:

- 1 pound wild caught large shrimp, peeled
- ¼ cup lemon juice
- 2 tbsp olive oil
- ¼ tsp ground pepper
- ¼ tsp salt

How to prepare:

Place the shrimp onto skewers.

Preheat a non-stick flat baking pan over medium-high heat.

In a small bowl, mix the olive oil, lemon juice, pepper and salt. Then baste the shrimp skewers.

Put the shrimp skewers onto the baking cook for 5 minutes and then turn and cook for additional 5 minutes.

Remove shrimp skewers and place on a serving plate. Allow to cool and serve.

Nutritional facts:

Calories: 230, Fat: 18g, Carbs: 4g, Protein: 21g

41.   Quinoa and its Friends

Description:

Quinoa is rich in cancer fighting compounds, including polyphenols and saponins. Combined with garlic and peppers, we have here a delicious, and very healthy meal.

Ingredients:

- 2 cups uncooked quinoa
- 2 tbsp olive oil
- 1 shallot, minced
- 2 cloves garlic, minced
- 1 red pepper, diced
- 1 yellow pepper, diced
- 2 cups broth, chicken or beef per choice
- 2 tbsp parsley, chopped

How to prepare:

Heat the olive oil in a large saucepan over medium-high heat.

Add the minced shallot and minced garlic, and cook for 3 minutes, stirring occasionally.

Add the parsley, quinoa and yellow and red peppers, and heat for 1 minute, stirring occasionally.

Add the broth, stir and cover saucepan.

Allow to cook for 15 minutes, checking for the quinoa to be tender.

Remove saucepan from heat and allow to cool, then serve.

Nutritional facts:

Calories: 216, Fat 7g, Carbs 32g, Protein 9g

42.   Trusty Watercress Salad

Description:

Watercress, which makes a nice addition to salads and sandwiches, is an anti-cancer food par excellence as it contains a compound called phenethyl isothiocyanate. This chemical has strong cancer fighting powers and for this reason, it is suggested that eating fresh watercress often can reduce the risk of cancer.

Ingredients:

- 1 tbsp lime juice
- ¼ cup olive oil
- 1 tsp minced fresh ginger root
- 1 tsp organic sugar
- 2 ½ cups cubed watermelon
- 2 cups of chopped watercress
- 2 ½ cups cubed cantaloupe
- ¼ cup toasted and sliced almonds

How to prepare:

In a large bowl, whisk together ginger, lime juice, and sugar. Slowly season with salt and pepper and pour the olive oil.

Add watercress, cantaloupe, and watermelon to large bowl and mix lightly. Sprinkle with sliced almonds and serve.

Nutritional facts:

Calories 274, Fat: 21g, Carbs: 22g, Protein 16g

ADDITIONAL TITLES FROM THIS AUTHOR

70 Effective Meal Recipes to Prevent and Solve Being Overweight: Burn Fat Fast by Using Proper Dieting and Smart Nutrition

By

Joe Correa CSN

48 Acne Solving Meal Recipes: The Fast and Natural Path to Fixing Your Acne Problems in Less Than 10 Days!

By

Joe Correa CSN

41 Alzheimer's Preventing Meal Recipes: Reduce or Eliminate Your Alzheimer's Condition in 30 Days or Less!

By

Joe Correa CSN

70 Effective Breast Cancer Meal Recipes: Prevent and Fight Breast Cancer with Smart Nutrition and Powerful Foods

By

Joe Correa CSN

www.ingramcontent.com/pod-product-compliance
Lightning Source LLC
Chambersburg PA
CBHW030252030426
42336CB00009B/354